Ítalo Câmara de Almeida

Bovine female reproduction

AF293031

Ítalo Câmara de Almeida

Bovine female reproduction

Physiology and fixed-time artificial insemination

Imprint
Any brand names and product names mentioned in this book are subject to trademark, brand or patent protection and are trademarks or registered trademarks of their respective holders. The use of brand names, product names, common names, trade names, product descriptions etc. even without a particular marking in this work is in no way to be construed to mean that such names may be regarded as unrestricted in respect of trademark and brand protection legislation and could thus be used by anyone.

Cover image: www.ingimage.com

This book is a translation from the original published under ISBN 978-613-9-72492-5.

Publisher:
Sciencia Scripts
is a trademark of
Dodo Books Indian Ocean Ltd. and OmniScriptum S.R.L publishing group

120 High Road, East Finchley, London, N2 9ED, United Kingdom
Str. Armeneasca 28/1, office 1, Chisinau MD-2012, Republic of Moldova, Europe
Printed at: see last page
ISBN: 978-620-7-74010-9

1

Foreword

This book is designed to help interested people understand the basic principles of the reproductive physiology of the female bovine, as well as one of the most widespread reproductive biotechnologies in Brazil, fixed-time artificial insemination. The book is easy to understand and a good read makes learning easier, takes less time and the knowledge is retained forever.

This book has been based on scientific studies published in the field, and it's not just about making sure that the information it contains is correct, it's also about making sure that people can understand it. There will always be room for debate regarding the topics in this book, as constant changes and technological advances are taking place in the field of veterinary medicine and bovine reproduction.

Happy reading!

SUMMARY

INTRODUCTION

Cattle farming plays an important role in Brazil's economic performance and job creation, making a fundamental contribution to its development. According to the Brazilian Institute of Geography and Statistics - IBGE (2011), Brazil has the second largest cattle herd in the world, second only to India. It is the largest exporter of meat of this species and, in 2010, total milk production was 30.7 million litres, making it the fifth largest producer in the world.

Brazil is the fifth largest milk producer in the world and is growing at an annual rate of 4 per cent, higher than all the countries that occupy the top spots, and accounts for 66 per cent of the total volume of milk produced in the countries that make up Mercosur (EMBRAPA, 2010).

The importance of dairy farming in Brazil's economic performance and job creation is fundamental. Total milk production in 2004 was 23.5 billion litres, generating revenues of approximately 12 billion reais. The primary sector involves around 5 million people, including the 1.3 million dairy farmers (ASSIS et al., 2005).

The introduction of reproductive biotechnologies in dairy farming has boosted the sector's productivity, increasing producers' income, providing genetic improvement for the herd, increasing the number of calvings and reducing the interval between calvings. Together with the use of reproductive biotechnologies, there are other factors of paramount importance for increasing herd productivity, such as: herd health (MONTEZUMA JR, 2001), nutrition and body condition (FERREIRA, 2000), lactation and productive management (MONTEZUMA JR, 2001).

Thus, there is a great deal of complexity surrounding dairy farming in order to achieve good reproductive efficiency in the herd. However, for some time now strategies have been used to increase the pregnancy rate, reduce the calving interval and increase the percentage of females in the herd.

In this context, we find Fixed-Term Artificial Insemination (FTAI), which allows cows to calve strategically, forming standardised and homogenous batches, reducing the occurrence of reproductive problems and the interval between calving, and improving the genetic quality of the animals (SÁ FILHO et al., 2006).

In view of its importance to the economy, there is a need to carry out studies on the use of FTAI in order to achieve greater efficiency in applied reproductive biotechnology and its viability. To this end, there is a need to inform professionals, students, producers and rural workers, detailing all the steps required to implement the Fixed-Term Artificial Insemination technique, in order to avoid losses and discouragement caused by negative results.

Farming in Brazil is of significant economic and social importance. The zootechnical and economic indices obtained in the country are still low when compared to other countries in the world, with a loss of competitiveness. One of the aggravating factors is the low use of available biotechnologies to increase the reproductive capacity of animals. As a result, we have herds with poor genetic quality and low production efficiency.

The practice of IATF is still used in small numbers, given Brazil's large herd. There is a need to improve the application of this technique in order to obtain better results and popularise its use.

In order to implement a reproductive programme of this size, it is necessary to inform professionals, students and producers, through lectures, training courses and book launches, of all the steps required to implement the Fixed-Time Artificial Insemination technique. The aim of this study was therefore to carry out a study on the reproductive physiology of female cattle and the use of hormonal fixed-time artificial insemination protocols to optimise the production system.

CHAPTER 1: Reproductive Physiology of the Bovine Female

1 Hormonal Interactions

Cow reproduction is controlled by interactions between the hypothalamus, the pituitary gland and the reproductive tract. The hypothalamus is located at the base of the brain and is made up of groups of nerve cell bodies. These cell bodies are responsible for producing hormones such as gonadotropin-releasing hormone (GnRH) and oxytocin (SENGER, 2003).

GnRH's target organ is the pituitary gland, located below the hypothalamus and responsible for producing the main reproductive hormones follicle stimulating hormone (FSH) and luteinising hormone (LH). FSH is mainly responsible for stimulating follicle development, and LH for participating in the final growth of the follicle until ovulation, causing ovulation and transforming the follicle into a corpus luteum (SENGER, 2003).

GnRH is responsible for controlling the sequence of events that occur in the oestrus cycle, it stimulates the release of FSH and LH from the pituitary. FSH and LH stimulate the ovary to produce waves of follicular development (ARIAS et al., 2006).

There are three stages to a follicular wave: recruitment, selection and dominance. Each follicular wave begins with the recruitment of a group of small follicles, then the recruited follicles go through a selection process where most undergo atresia and one becomes dominant. Follicle development results in increasing levels of oestrogen and inhibin. Both hormones inhibit the release of FSH, resulting in the atresia of the other follicles in the group (ARIAS et al., 2006).

As the dominant follicle grows, it produces more oestrogen. When the level of estrogen reaches a threshold, it triggers a wave of GnRH, which stimulates the release of peak LH, which leads the follicle to ovulate and release the egg. This can only happen when there is no progesterone (P_4), produced by the CL, as it has an inhibitory effect on the GnRH wave. Oestrogen is also responsible for the behavioural signs of oestrus (SENGER, 2003).

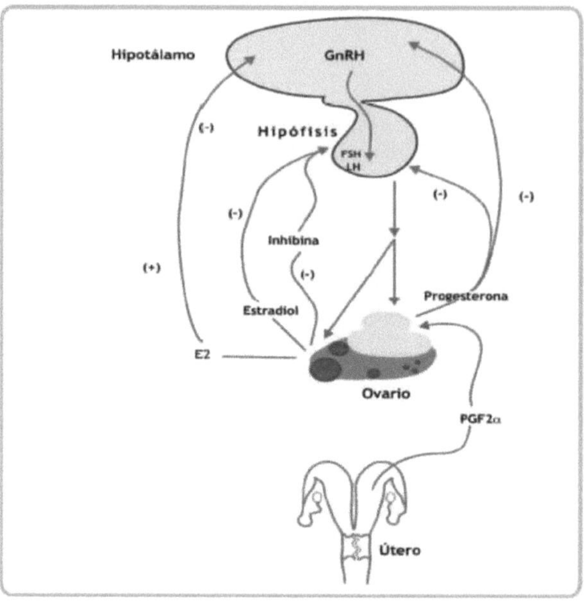

Figure 5: Hormonal interactions in the control of the oestrus cycle (ALMERAYA, 2010).

Bovine females normally have 2 to 3 follicular waves in each oestrus cycle, which can vary from 1 to 4 waves. The dominant follicles that develop during the luteal phase undergo atresia. After lysis of the corpus luteum, the oestrous cycle enters the follicular phase. During the follicular phase, the dominant follicle continues its development until ovulation. After ovulation, LH causes luteinisation of the ruptured follicle cells to form the corpus luteum. CL is responsible for producing progesterone, which prepares and maintains the uterus for pregnancy. P4 is fundamental in controlling the oestrus cycle, as it has an inhibitory effect on the release of the GnRH wave. Without the GnRH wave, there is no LH peak and oestrus and ovulation do not occur. However, there is still a basal release of GnRH allowing follicle development (BÓ et al., 2000).

If the cow is not pregnant, the uterus releases prostaglandin (PGF2a), which results in the lysis of the corpus luteum. Lysis of the corpus luteum removes the inhibitory effect of progesterone on the release of the GnRH surge, resulting in the release of GnRH stimulating the LH surge that matures the dominant follicle (SENGER, 2003).

1.2 Estral Cycle

Puberty is the process of reproductive acquisition, and its onset depends on the specific ability of the hypothalamus to produce sufficient quantities of GnRH to promote and maintain gametogenesis (SENGER, 2003). The reproductive activity of the female bovine begins at puberty, when the animal is around 40 to 45 per cent of the weight of an adult animal. The female bovine is considered a continuous polyestrus, i.e. the oestrus cycle is not interrupted by seasonal changes. This cycle lasts an average of 21-22 days in adult cows and 20 days in heifers, and can vary between 18-24 days (ARIAS et al., 2006).

After puberty, the female enters a period of reproductive cyclicity that continues throughout her life. The oestrus cycle consists of a series of events that begin with oestrus and end with the subsequent oestrus. They continue throughout the female's adult life and are interrupted by pregnancy, illness, inadequate nutrition or stressful environmental conditions. These events are responsible for morphophysiological changes in the female genital tract that reappear periodically according to a well-defined rhythm for each species. These changes are dependent on the cyclical production of ovarian hormones, oestrogen and progesterone, which in turn are under the control of pituitary gonadotrophic hormones - follicle stimulating hormone and luteinising hormone (SENGER, 2003).

The oestrus cycle can be divided into two distinct phases which are named according to the predominant structure present in the ovary during each phase of the cycle. These divisions of the cycle are the follicular phase and the luteal phase. The follicular phase is the period from the regression of the corpus luteum until ovulation. This phase is generally short, and the dominant ovarian structure is the growing follicles which mainly produce oestradiol. The luteal phase is the period after ovulation until the corpus luteum regresses. It is longer, and the dominant structure in the ovary is the corpus luteum which produces progesterone (SENGER, 2003).

With regard to the changes that occur during the oestrus cycle, four stages can be distinguished: proestrus, oestrus, meta-estrus and diestrus (SENGER, 2003). Proestrus is the period that immediately precedes oestrus. It lasts around 3 days and begins with degenerative changes in the LC. In this phase, general proliferative phenomena occur. The ovarian follicles increase in volume due to the action of pituitary gonadotrophins and under the action of the estrogen produced by these follicles, the endometrium and vaginal walls thicken with an increase in blood supply. It is characterised by a major endocrine transition, moving from a period of progesterone dominance to one of estrogen dominance. The gonadotropins FSH and LH are the hormones responsible for this transition, and it is during proestrus that follicles are recruited for ovulation and the female reproductive system prepares to start oestrus (SENGER, 2003).

Oestrus is the best known stage of the oestrus cycle, as it is characterised by sexually receptive behaviour. Oestrus lasts approximately 18 hours in European breeds, but shorter periods are observed in Zebu breeds. The presence of a bull can shorten this phase and nutritional and/or environmental conditions tend to suppress signs of oestrus due to reduced oestrogen secretion (SENGER, 2003).

At this stage, follicle growth is at its peak and the general proliferative phenomena that began in proestrus are emphasised. This phase is of great practical importance, as the external signs of oestrus become noticeable, such as restlessness and contact-seeking (mounting other females), frequent mooing, elimination of mucus from the vagina, hyperemia of the vaginal vestibule and, as oestrus progresses, the female begins to lordose (arching her back for copulation) and begins to accept the male (SENGER, 2003). Ovulation is an ovarian response to the secretion of 17-0 oestradiol and the pre-ovulatory peak of LH and occurs around 30 hours after the start of oestrus, i.e. between 10 and 12 hours after the end of oestrus.

Metaestrus is the period of hormonal transition from oestrogen dominance to progesterone dominance, i.e. the period between ovulation and the formation of the CL. P4 will cause secretory changes in the endometrium, cervix and vagina. This phase lasts approximately 34 days (SENGER, 2003).

Diestrus is the longest stage of the estrous cycle, lasting approximately 10 to 13 days and characterised by a period of sexual inactivity. In this stage the LC is fully functional and P4 production is high, blocking the hypothalamic-pituitary axis for pulsatile releases of FSH and LH. The rise in P4 prepares the uterus for the development of the initial embryo and eventually its hatching and nidation of the conceptus in the endometrium (SENGER, 2003).

At the end of diestrus, around the 17th day of the oestrus cycle, if an embryo has not implanted, the endometrium secretes PGF2a which lyses the corpus luteum (luteolysis) and induces the process of involution of the CL, thus restarting a new cycle (SENGER, 2003).

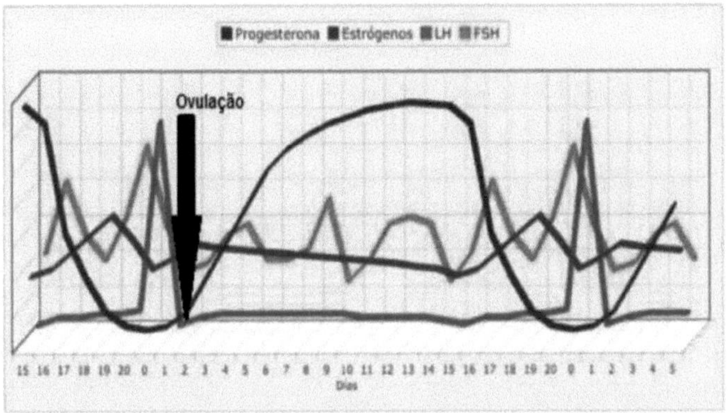

Figure 6 Schematic of an oestrus cycle and its hormonal relationship with FSH, LH, progesterone and oestrogen (ARIAS et al., 2006).

1.3 Follicular Dynamics

Follicular dynamics is a process of follicular growth and regression of antral follicles that leads to the development of a pre-ovulatory follicle, and occurs continuously throughout the oestrus cycle. The process of follicular development occurs in a wave system (SENGER, 2003).

Waves of follicular growth and development occur during a single oestrus cycle in cows, with the pre-ovulatory follicle being derived from the last wave. Follicular growth waves occur at various physiological stages experienced by a bovine female, such as during an entire estrous cycle during pregnancy in prepubertal heifers and in the postpartum period (BÓ et al.,2000). During the follicular wave, there are distinct phases: recruitment, selection and dominance.

Recruitment is the start of the follicular wave, through a minimal gonadotrophic stimulus, sufficient to allow progress towards ovulation. This phase lasts 2 to 3 days and is characterised by the simultaneous growth of several FSH-sensitive follicles (ARIAS et al., 2006). At the start of the oestrus cycle, a group of follicles is recruited from a *pool of* small antral follicles (2-4 mm). The association between the FSH surge and the emergence of a new follicular wave has been confirmed regardless of the stage of the oestrus cycle, and has been demonstrated in heifers aged 6 to 8 months, during pregnancy and in the postpartum period. Some factors control the increase and decrease in circulating FSH concentrations. Inhibin, which is one of the components of follicular fluid, has an inhibitory effect on FSH and follicular growth (SENGER, 2003).

At the end of the recruitment stage, the selection phase begins, which will allow the number of follicles that continue to grow to be adjusted to the number of ovulations characteristic of each species (ARIAS, et al., 2006). In cows, a single follicle usually emerges from the group of recruited follicles and continues to grow, while other recruited follicles decrease in size and go into atresia. Dominance is the way in which the selected follicle, or dominant follicle (DF), inhibits the recruitment of a new group of follicles (ARIAS, et al., 2006).

Dominance is characterised by the growth of the FD, which is defined as the largest ovarian follicle (> 10 mm) that is recruited and selected during a follicular wave, while the others continue in the process of atresia. The activity of the FD is able to prevent the recruitment of other follicles in the ovary where, through a negative feedback mechanism, oestradiol (E_2) and inhibin, produced by the growing follicle (FD), decrease circulating FSH concentrations and thus prevent the appearance of a new wave of follicular growth. As circulating FSH levels fall, only follicles with a greater number of LH receptors are able to develop. These include the follicle destined to be the ovulatory follicle, which has the highest number of LH receptors of all the other (subordinate) follicles and can survive without FSH (BARUSELLI & MADUREIRA, 2000).

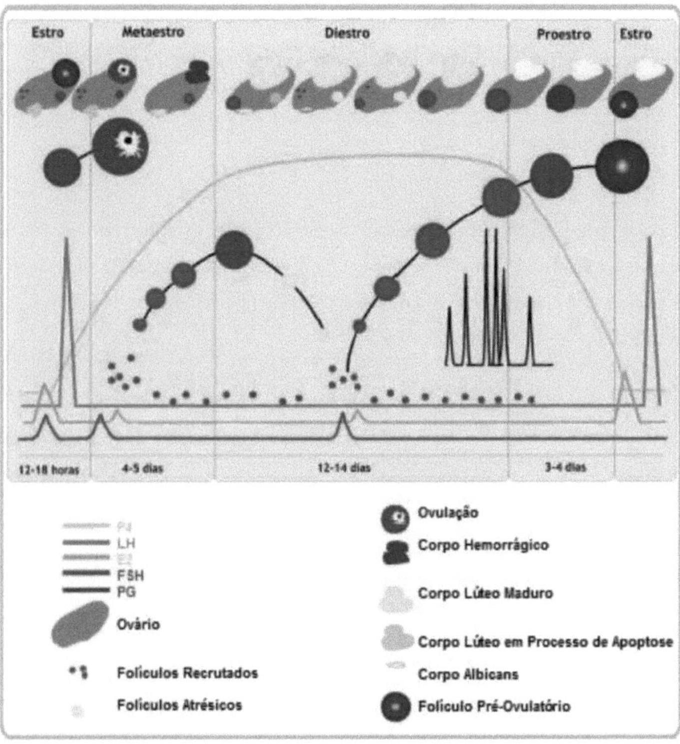

Figure 7. Diagram of two follicular waves in the bovine oestrus cycle, hormonal interaction and phases of the reproductive cycle (ALMERAYA, 2010).

The change in ovarian follicles during the oestrus cycle in cows is regulated by the concentration of P4 in the plasma, acting via negative feedback on LH secretion and that the low frequency of LH pulses characteristic of the luteal phase is not enough to maintain continuous growth and functional FD (ALMERAYA, 2010).

A good dominant follicle generates a functional CL, which is responsible for the length of the oestrus cycle, with luteolysis being the main factor for ovulation to occur. After luteolysis, there is a decrease in circulating concentrations of P4, which undoes the negative feedback with LH, from which point the frequency of LH pulses begins to increase, stimulating the final development of the dominant follicle. Under the influence of the increased frequency and low amplitude of LH pulses, the FD begins the pre-ovulatory growth phase, resulting in a subsequent increase in the production of androgens and oestrogens.

The increase in E2 production stimulates oestrus behaviour and causes a FSH/LH surge that is responsible for ovulation (BARUSELLI & MADUREIRA, 2000).

1.3 Service period (SP) and calving interval (PI)

The service period, or days open, is defined as the period (in days) between calving and the first fertile conception confirmed by the cow's pregnancy. This index helps to assess the nutritional and health status of the animals and their return to ovarian activity, the efficiency of heat observation and AI or the sexual behaviour and seminal quality of the sire.

The calving interval is the period in months from the date of the previous calving to the current calving. It is directly related to SP. Analysing this index provides an overall assessment of the herd's reproductive performance. As the gestation period in cattle does not vary much, on average 285 days, PI, considered the final indicator of a herd's reproductive performance, is directly related to SP. In this sense, to obtain an IP of 12 months (ideal), the SP should not exceed 85 days.

1.4 Reproductive Efficiency

Reproductive efficiency is one of the main factors influencing dairy herd productivity. Nutritional and health factors and problems in identifying oestrus contribute to a delayed return to postpartum ovarian activity, a longer service period and calving interval, a reduction in the lactation period and a lower production of calves per year and during their lifetime. Consequently, production costs are increased by keeping animals with low production in the herd.

Poor reproductive performance leads to lower milk and calf production, higher maintenance costs for dry cows and higher culling rates. Reproductive efficiency is therefore one of the factors that most contributes to improving the performance and profitability of dairy herds (GROHN; RAJALA - SCHULTZ, 2000).

Therefore, reproductive efficiency is reduced when a lactating cow fails to have a normal oestrus cycle between 50 and 60 days postpartum. The factors considered to limit profitability are low conception rates (CT) and pregnancy per artificial insemination (P/IA) (SARTORI, 2007).

Some nutritional, health and reproductive management problems, such as failure to detect oestrus, puerperal and metabolic diseases, partly influence the herd's reproductive performance and, indirectly, milk production per day of the cow's life (BARBOSA, 2009).

As a result of the reduction in the reproductive performance of the dairy herd on the property, there will be a lower production of milk and calves, adding to the costs of maintaining dry cows and a higher discard rate (BARBOSA, 2009).

1.5 Factors Affecting Reproductive Efficiency

Infertility can be a serious problem, especially in high-producing dairy cows. During the postpartum period, there needs to be a rapid and trauma-free involution of the uterus accompanied by a rapid resumption of normal ovarian activity, followed by accurate oestrus detection with a high conception rate (BARUSELLI, 2007).

1.6.1 Stress

Environmental stress such as climate, high population density or excessive management during the pre-coital period can depress oestrus, ovulation and lutein function (HAFEZ, HAFEZ 2003).

Heat stress compromises reproductive events by reducing the expression of oestrus behaviour, altering follicular development and inhibiting embryonic development (HANSEN et al., 2000). Holstein cows exposed to heat stress, with an average daily maximum temperature >29°C from 20-50 days before artificial insemination, had a lower pregnancy rate (23% vs 31.3%) than cows not exposed to this environmental condition (p<0.001) (CHEBEL et al., 2004).

The rate of failure to detect oestrus reaches 75-80% in the hottest months of the year, when the greatest effects of heat stress are observed, as the high temperature reduces both the duration of oestrus and the number of mounts. Heat stress can also reduce TC by 10% or more during this period of the year (HANSEN, 2000).

During the peripartum period, the focus should be on reducing animal stress. Increased stress during this phase is positively correlated with an increased incidence of postpartum diseases, especially retained placenta. In addition to retained placenta, delayed uterine involution and postpartum uterine infections are related to increased PI in cows (SHELDON et al., 2000). Hormonal treatments with exogenous PG in the immediate postpartum period can potentially speed up uterine recovery and, consequently, increase the reproductive efficiency of cows (ZANCHET, 2005).

1.6.2 Ovulation failure

Different forms of stress can lead to ovulation failure, making it important to consider when evaluating causes of infertility in dairy herds. According to Lopez - Gatius et al. (2005), there is a 3.9 times greater chance of failure occurring in hot seasons compared to cold seasons that year. Demétrio et al. (2007), working with lactating Holstein cows, found that of 387 oestrus manifestations after PG application, 84.8% (328/387) had CL on day 7, i.e. 15.2% of the cows failed to ovulate. According to Sartori (2007), because heifers suffer less from climatological changes, they don't suffer changes in ovulation rates (OT) during the hottest months of the year.

1.6.3 Presence of Short Cycle

One factor to be concerned about when dealing with cows at the beginning of the postpartum period is the occurrence of short cycles (8 to 12 days), which is characterised by a premature regression of the CL resulting from the first postpartum ovulation, causing a change in the cycle (SÁ FILHO et al., 2006). This is probably due to the premature release of PG by the endometrium. In this way, the uterus in the postpartum period produces PG in greater quantities and, when the first ovulation occurs, with no previous exposure of the uterus to $P4$, this high concentration of PG smoothes the LC, at the same time as it becomes responsive, which ends up resulting in a short luteal phase. According to Sá Filho et al. (2006), when comparing postpartum cows that received P4 implants with cows that did not receive $P4$ implants, it was observed that there was no premature regression of the LC in the group that received the implants, while in the animals that did not receive the implants, all showed premature regression of the LC.

1.6.4 Nutrition and Metabolic Diseases

Among many other factors that affect the reproductive performance of dairy cows, nutritional management has the greatest impact, with energy being the main nutrient required for the reproduction of bovine females. It is important to emphasise that in relation to protein, both deficiency and excess can harm reproductive performance (FERREIRA, 2000).

Insufficient intake of quality nutrients in adequate quantity is one of the main causes of infertility in dairy herds, inhibiting ovarian activity, delaying puberty and prolonging postpartum anestrus (FERREIRA, 2000).

Inhibition of ovarian activity occurs due to alterations in endocrine mechanisms, with the effect of suppressing the release and secretion of gonadotropins, resulting in a reduction in the pulsatile secretion of LH (WILTBANK et al., 2002).

According to Wiltbank *et al.* (2002), this alteration in the secretion of gonadotropins reduces the maximum diameter of the FD and the duration of the follicular growth wave. As a result, the energy ingested by the animal is prioritised for the vital functions of maintenance and milk production, leaving the reproductive functions of the animal lacking.

1.6.5 Negative Energy Balance (NEB)

BEN can be defined as the deficit found after subtracting the net energy intake provided by the feed minus the net energy needed for maintenance and milk production. This is due to the fact that the animals reach peak production before the maximum dry matter intake (BARBOSA, 2009).

Considered a key factor in restoring postpartum ovarian activity, pituitary LH secretion is reduced in primiparous cows that are in BEN (YAVAS; WALTON, 2000).

Postpartum anestrus, caused among other things by BEN, can reduce reproductive efficiency by delaying the first service, since cows that do not show oestrus in the first 30 days postpartum require more services per conception with a greater risk of being discarded (THATCHER et al., 2001).

1.6.6 Body Condition Score (BCS)

Each cow has an ideal body mass for optimum fertility, and when this mass declines or increases beyond certain limits, reproduction is affected. There is a minimum weight below which the cow will not conceive or will stop cycling, which would occur when the cow loses 20 to 30 per cent of its adult weight (FERREIRA, 2000).

According to Montiel and Ahuja (2005), assessing the herd's ECC and nutrition is an extremely important tool in reproductive management. It is common for cows to be ready for AI when they approach their lactation peak (around 60 days postpartum). As a result, BEN and ECC are declining and evaluating the latter in the period prior to entering service is excellent information for prognosticating cow fertility (BANOS et al., 2004).

Meneghetti and Vasconcelos (2008), evaluating the relationship between ECC and the response to an FTAI protocol in primiparous beef cows, observed that there was a positive effect of ECC on the synchronisation rate of these cows and also observed that animals with lower ECC had a smaller follicle diameter at the time of FTAI. Follicles are affected by the animal's body condition, with a consequent decrease in the number of dominant follicles.

The determination of ECC is subjective and is based on visual observation and/or palpation of specific areas of the animal's body surface (ribs, dorsal and caudal region, hips, tail insertion, etc.) in order to consider the amounts of adipose tissue deposits and muscle mass, and is considered a very practical and useful assessment for determining the nutritional level of each animal (MACIEL, 2006).

Cows must be observed carefully to assess their body reserves. Some methods involve palpating certain areas, requiring more appropriate restraint of the animals. The most commonly used scale in dairy herds is the one that ranges from 1 to 5 (MACIEL, 2006), where 1 is for an extremely thin cow and 5 is for an extremely fat cow.

1.6.7 Dominant Follicle Diameter (FD)

Even when a hormonal protocol based on progesterone and oestradiol is carried out in dairy cattle, in some animals there is no dominant follicle and ovulation does not occur. The lack of a dominant follicle is a determining factor in why ovulation does not occur (BURKE et al., 2001).

According to Burke et al. (2001), the ovulatory potential and development of the luteal phase in lactating or anestrous Holstein cattle is due to the maturity and ideal diameter of the dominant follicle on the day the progesterone implant is removed. In the study presented here, it was noted that cows with a larger follicle diameter (13.8 ± 0.4 mm) ovulated in their entirety (100%), while those with a smaller diameter (9.0 ± 0.6 mm) had a reduced number of ovulations (50%).

In an experiment, Sartori et al. (2001) used lactating Dutch cows and, using ultrasound, it was observed in these animals that the dominant follicles with diameters of 7 - 8.5 and 10 mm did not ovulate even when they were given LH at concentrations of 4, 24 and 40 mg. Therefore, 75 per cent of follicles with a diameter of 10 mm and 100 per cent of follicles with a diameter of 12 mm ovulated at doses of 40 and 4 mg respectively. These results prove that in *Bos taurus* cattle, dominant follicles with a diameter greater than 10 mm have a greater ovulatory capacity when subjected to hormonal protocols than follicles with smaller diameters.

According to Gimenes et al. (2008), *Bos indicus* cattle have dominant follicles with smaller diameters when compared to *Bos taurus*. *In* this sense, the likelihood of ovulation can be improved in hormonal protocols by using animals with larger diameter dominant follicles.

CHAPTER 2: Fixed-Term Artificial Insemination

2.1 Artificial Insemination (AI)

Artificial insemination was the first major reproductive biotechnology applied to the genetic improvement of domestic animals. In cattle it is a well-established technique today and has been implemented in combination with genetic selection programmes, which include progeny testing and performance evaluation (BARBOSA, et al., 2009).

There is a long list of benefits that can be obtained through the use of AI, such as: greater weight gain, greater precocity, higher milk production, better conformation, herd standardisation, control of sexually transmitted diseases and a reduction in the cost of replacing bulls (GOUFERT, 2008). But the main advantage of AI is directly linked to the process of genetic improvement, obtaining animals with greater production and reproduction potential (BARUSELLI, 2007).

Work carried out in Brazil and in various countries has shown that the biggest limitation to the use of AI is the reduction in the herd's service rate, which subsequently compromises reproductive efficiency when compared to the use of natural mating. Estrus detection failures associated with the low cyclicity rate observed in postpartum cows are limiting factors that prevent AI from providing reproductive efficiency comparable to the use of bulls (GOUFERT, 2008).

The main obstacle to AI lies in heat detection: when few cows are detected in heat, there are significant losses in the herd's reproductive efficiency, thus jeopardising the technique. This impairment is even greater in *Bos indicus* (zebu) herds, whose reproductive behaviour has particular characteristics, such as short-lived oestrus, manifesting mainly at night (BARUSELLI, 2007).

According to ANUALPEC (2004), 80% of breeding cows in Brazil have zebu blood and are mostly raised on pasture, significantly compromising the heat detection rate and the efficiency of AI programmes.

In Brazil, it is estimated that only 10% of females of reproductive age are inseminated, and according to the Brazilian Artificial Insemination Association (2009), just over 9 million doses of semen were sold this year.

2.2 Fixed Time Artificial Insemination (FTAI)

According to Barros (2001), in the last decade, a better understanding of the physiology of ovarian follicle growth has led to the development of hormonal treatments capable of controlling the timing of ovulation. This has made it possible to use fixed-time artificial insemination (FTAI), i.e. AI at a predetermined time, without the need to observe oestrus.

IATF involves the use of hormonal substances to synchronise and induce oestrus and ovulation. Various hormones are used to induce puberty in heifers and synchronise oestrus in beef and dairy cows and heifers, thus increasing the reproductive efficiency of these animals (CASTILHO et al., 2000; BRAGANÇA et al., 2004; VOGG et al., 2004). According to Thatcher et al. (2001) follicle growth can be induced using different hormones such as P_4, E2 and a combination of these, as well as GnRH and its analogues.

According to Goufert (2008), there are several IATF protocols published by different researchers and companies, but they all follow three basic principles:

1. <u>Follicular wave synchronisation</u>: the aim is to get all treated cows to start growing ovarian follicles at the same time;

2. <u>Controlling follicular growth and blocking ovulation</u>: using pharmacological methods, the level of progesterone is kept high during the follicular growth and dominance phase, and then progesterone levels fall in all the females so that they all start the preovulatory phase together;

3. <u>Ovulation synchronisation</u>: through the use of drugs capable of triggering the ovulatory process, it is possible for the vast majority of treated females to ovulate at a known time, allowing inseminations to be carried out in good time and subject to prior scheduling.

IATF is a reproductive biotechnique that makes it possible to concentrate AI and calving cows at desirable times within production systems. There are programmes that use IATF without the need for oestrus detection and they directly help to use this biotechnology (BARUSELLI and SENEDA, 2004) by optimising time, labour and financial resources, allowing a greater number of animals to become pregnant with AI.

The advantages of IATF include the fact that it eliminates the need to observe oestrus; it avoids inseminating cows out of time, reducing the waste of semen, material and labour; it induces cyclicity in cows in transitional anestrus, making it possible to inseminate these females; it reduces the interval between calving, increasing the number of calves born; it makes it possible to schedule inseminations in a short period of time; concentrating the return of oestrus of failed females in the first fixed-time insemination, making it easier to diagnose oestrus when breeding; enabling high pregnancy rates at the start of the breeding season; concentrating labour, reducing the number of overtime hours spent by technicians and inseminators; reducing the disposal and replacement cost of herd matrices; reducing investment in the purchase of bulls (BARUSELLI et al., 2004). In view of all the results offered by the IATF technique, it is possible to achieve major advances in dairy productivity by using it.

2.3 Factors that interfere with Fixed-Term Artificial Insemination

Monitoring the IATF programme by a veterinarian is extremely important, as only this professional will be able to analyse the herd's health, nutritional and reproductive condition, which are fundamental factors if the programmes are to achieve the expected results.

Body condition is a relevant factor to consider, as there is a clear correlation between ECC and the results obtained in IATF programmes.

Figure 8. ECC and IATF pregnancy results (CUTAIA et al., 2003).

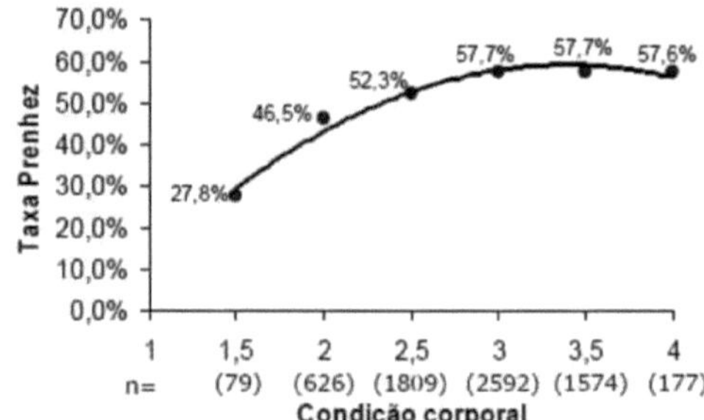

Another factor that influences the results is the high level of milk production associated with high nutritional intake and the corresponding metabolic activity, which affects reproductive efficiency and translates into a reduction in pregnancies after AI. High-producing Holstein cows have short-lived oestrus due to a lower circulating concentration of oestradiol as a result of the increased hepatic metabolism of this steroid (WILTBANK, 2006). The high level of milk production also compromises the initial luteal function, thus affecting early embryonic development (BARUSELLI, 2007).

According to Neves (2010), heat stress affects sperm quality and, on the day of oestrus and the days corresponding to the first embryonic divisions, results in gestational losses.

The quality of the semen used is also an important factor in the variability of the results of IATF programmes. It is essential that the quality of the semen to be used is previously analysed for fertility in order to avoid unpleasant surprises in the results.

According to Goufert (2008), other fundamental precautions for IATF programmes to achieve adequate results are:

- avoid failure in the application of the drugs by handling the hormones properly, respecting the recommended times and doses;

- carry out the semen thawing and applicator assembly phases with the necessary care;

- work with well-trained inseminators and change the inseminator every 30 animals inseminated, in order to avoid fatigue and a drop in indices;

- control of the execution of the programme with spreadsheets, reliably identifying that all the females have gone through all the stages of the programme.

2.4 Hormonal interactions in the female bovine

Cow reproduction is controlled by interactions between the hypothalamus, the pituitary gland and the reproductive tract. The hypothalamus is located at the base of the brain and is made up of groups of nerve cell bodies. These cell bodies are responsible for producing hormones such as gonadotropin-releasing hormone (GnRH) and oxytocin (SENGER, 2003).

GnRH's target organ is the pituitary gland. Located below the hypothalamus, it is responsible for producing the main reproductive hormones: follicle stimulating hormone (FSH) and luteinising hormone (LH). FSH is mainly responsible for stimulating follicle development, and LH for participating in the final growth of the follicle until ovulation, causing ovulation and transforming the follicle into a corpus luteum. GnRH, responsible for controlling the sequence of events that occur in the oestrus cycle, stimulates the release of FSH and LH, which in turn stimulate the ovary to produce waves of follicular development (SENGER, 2003).

According to Ginther et al. (2003), follicular development in cattle takes place through follicular waves divided into: recruitment, selection and dominance. Each follicular wave begins with the recruitment of a small group of follicles (follicular emergence), then the recruited follicles go through a selection process where the majority undergo atresia (subordinate follicles) and one continues its development (dominant follicle - DF), this process is called follicular divergence. The development of the dominant follicle results in increased levels of oestrogen and inhibin, both of which inhibit the release of FSH, resulting in the atresia of the other follicles in the group.

As the dominant follicle grows, it produces more oestrogen. When estrogen concentrations reach a threshold, a wave of GnRH is triggered which stimulates the release of peak LH, which leads the follicle to ovulate and release the oocyte. This only happens when there is no progesterone (P4), produced by the corpus luteum (CL), as it has an inhibitory effect on the GnRH wave. Oestrogen is also responsible for the behavioural signs of oestrus (SENGER, 2003).

The corpus luteum is responsible for producing progesterone, which prepares and maintains the uterus for pregnancy. It is fundamental in controlling the oestrus cycle, as it has an inhibitory effect on the release of the GnRH wave. Without this wave, there is no LH peak and oestrus and ovulation do not occur. However, there is still a basal release of GnRH, thus allowing follicle development (BÓ et al., 2000).

If the cow is not pregnant, the uterus releases prostaglandin (PGF2a), which results in the lysis of the corpus luteum. Lysis of the corpus luteum removes the inhibitory effect of progesterone on the release of the GnRH surge, resulting in the release of GnRH stimulating the LH surge that matures the dominant follicle (SENGER, 2003).

2.5 Fixed Time Artificial Insemination - FTAI

Artificial insemination (AI) was the first major reproductive biotechnology applied to the genetic improvement of domestic animals. In cattle, it is a well-established technique today and has been implemented in combination with genetic selection programmes, which include progeny testing and performance evaluation (BARBOSA et al., 2011). However, the main obstacle to AI is heat detection. When few cows are detected in heat, there are significant losses in the herd's reproductive efficiency, jeopardising AI. This impairment is even greater in *Bos indicus* (zebu) herds, whose reproductive behaviour has particular characteristics, such as short-lived oestrus, manifested mainly at night (NEVES et al., 2010).

A better understanding of the physiology of ovarian follicle growth has led to the development of hormonal treatments capable of controlling the timing of ovulation, thus enabling the use of IATF, i.e. artificial insemination (AI) of animals at a predetermined time, without the need to observe oestrus. The aim of hormonal protocols applied to heifers or cows is for a greater number of animals to conceive in a shorter period of time (BARUSELLI et al., 2004) - usually at the start of the reproductive season, in addition to maximising the benefits and genetic gain from artificial insemination.

According to Severo (2009), the use of IATF programmes has numerous advantages: it eliminates the service of observing oestrus, making farm management easier; it synchronises and induces the animals' cyclicity; it reduces the effects of the environment and breastfeeding; it allows for rapid genetic improvement of the herd by using bulls with known and proven genetic data for productive characteristics; it increases the number of calves born by reducing the interval between calving and reduces the service period, thus improving pregnancy rates.

IATF consists of using hormonal substances to synchronise and induce oestrus and ovulation. Various hormones are used to induce oestrus in heifers and synchronise oestrus in heifers and beef and dairy cows, thus increasing the reproductive efficiency of these animals (VOGG et al., 2004). Oestrus synchronisation and ovulation synchronisation occur in different ways. In this sense, there are basic prerequisites for using the different types of synchronisation, related to the use of different hormone treatments, the animal category that responds best to each type of synchronisation and the minimum critical points that must be respected in each situation (GOTTSCHALL et al., 2012).

Various protocols are described in the literature, which show varying results depending on the health and nutritional condition of the females. When choosing a protocol, the individual conditions of each herd must be analysed, as well as the cost/benefit ratio of its use (MORAES et al., 2001). These treatments, when appropriate and respectful of animal physiology, can be very attractive as they allow for rationalisation in the use of artificial insemination (AI).

According to Meneghetti et al. (2009), the main protocols developed must essentially meet the following objectives: 1) induce ovulation in bovine females, including those in anestrus; 2) allow artificial insemination without the need to detect oestrus (IATF); 3) synchronise the wave of follicular development; 4) increase the growth of the dominant follicle; 5) prevent premature luteolysis after synchronised ovulation, and 6) be low cost and have a pregnancy rate close to 50%.

However, it is important that the results presented from the use of these protocols are consistent and repeatable, enabling high pregnancy rates to be obtained in different locations and situations (SIQUEIRA et al., 2008). The efficient application of these therapies could then allow for greater synchronisation of ovulation, increasing the rate of animals observed in oestrus and also efficiency when using artificial insemination (BÓ et al., 2003).

2.5.1 Progesterone

Progesterone (P_4) is a hormone that regulates the functioning of the female reproductive system and is secreted by the lutein cells of the corpus luteum (CL). Like oestrogens, it is derived from cholesterol and is also secreted by the placenta, testicles and adrenal cortex in small quantities.

P4 concentrations remain high throughout the functional life of the CL, which is important for embryonic development and the maintenance of pregnancy, as well as blocking LH waves and ovulation (WOAD and ARMSTRONG, 2002).

The exogenous administration of P_4 used to induce and synchronise oestrus mimics its biological effects, including the suppression of oestrus, the inhibition of the pre-ovulatory LH peak - which simulates the lutein phase of the cycle - and the regulation of pulsatile LH secretion. This process leads to the occurrence of follicular waves and their development (LARSON and BALL, 1992), associated with follicular maturation and ovulation in the days following its use (ODDE, 1990), since the suppression of progestational treatment leads to the occurrence of the LH peak (KESNER et al., 1982).

In this sense, a large number of synthetic progestogens have been used in the practice of oestrus cycle synchronisation, such as: medroxyprogesterone acetate (MAP); chlormadinone acetate (CAP); melengestrol acetate (MGA) and flurogesterone acetate (FGA), which are very effective as oestrus synchronisers.

Initial attempts to synchronise oestrus in female cattle using progestogens were based on the understanding that P4 prevents the occurrence of oestrus and ovulation (CHRISTIAN et al., 1948) by acting on the hypothalamus and regulating the release of GnRH (MIHM and AUSTIN, 2002) and, consequently, LH. These attempts were based on treatment with progestogens for a prolonged period of 14 to 21 days, the time needed for luteolysis to occur naturally, which would be effective for synchronising oestrus. However, the fertility of this synchronised oestrus is reduced (ODDE, 1990), contrary to popular belief. This effect occurs because the use of progesterone for periods longer than 13 days leads to the formation of larger dominant follicles (CUSTER et al., 1994; KINDER, 1996) and reduced fertility. Low fertility can be attributed to the spontaneous maturation of the oocyte (breakdown of the germinal vesicle and expansion of the *cumulus),* present in the persistent follicle (REVAH and BUTLER, 1996).

To avoid these problems of follicular persistence, it is understood that treatment with progestogens should not be too prolonged. The continuous administration of progesterone for 5 to 9 days inhibits the release of LH, and when its supply is interrupted, a wave of LH capable of inducing the final growth of the pre-ovulatory follicle is triggered, culminating in ovulation (MORAES et al., 2001).

2.5.2 Estrogen

Oestradiol 170 (E2) is a hormone produced by the granulosa cells of growing follicles. They are substances derived from cholesterol and their immediate precursors are androstenedione and testosterone.

The tissue responses induced by estrogens include stimulation of endometrial glandular growth, stimulation of duct growth in the mammary gland, increased secretory activity of the uterine ducts, induction of sexual receptivity, regulation of LH and FSH secretion by the anterior pituitary gland, regulation of PGF_{2a} release by the non-pregnant and pregnant uterus and protein anabolism (SOUZA et al., 2011).

The endogenous E2 produced by ovarian follicles accentuates the amplitude of LH pulses during the follicular phase of the oestrus cycle by increasing LH-releasing hormone receptors in the anterior pituitary and the consequent increase in the oestrogenic capacity of pre-ovulatory follicles (STUMPF et al., 1989). This positive feedback mechanism between E2 and LH is critical in the process of final maturation of the ovulatory follicle, inducing oestrus behaviour and ovulation (FIKE et al., 1997).

The administration of exogenous E2 can stimulate or inhibit the release of gonadotropins, depending on the dose and blood concentrations of progesterone. At physiological doses and low progesterone concentrations, E2 stimulates the release of LH so that ovulation occurs. On the other hand, high doses of E2, in the presence of high concentrations of progesterone, block gonadotrophins, suppressing any dominant follicle that may lead to the emergence of a new follicular wave (BÓ et al., 2004; MADUREIRA et al., 2009).

E2 was introduced into oestrus synchronisation protocols with short exposure to progesterone in order to increase negative *feedback* to gonadotropins, allowing for better synchronisation of the follicular wave (YAVAS and WALTON, 2000). The administration of E2 at the beginning of the FTAI protocol, together with the insertion of the slow-release progesterone device, inhibits the secretion of both LH and FSH by negative feedback on the hypothalamic-pituitary axis (CLARKE, 1988; MARTINEZ et al., 2003).

Currently, several synthetic compounds that have the same biological activities as natural estrogens have been developed and are frequently used in reproductive programmes to synchronise follicular waves, ovulate the dominant follicle and induce oestrus. The most commonly used estrogens for this purpose are 17 P-estradiol (E2) and estradiol esters such as estradiol benzoate (BE), estradiol valerate (VE) and estradiol cypionate (CE). However, only the 17 P oestradiol molecule is biologically active. Estradiol esters (BE, VE and CE) need to release 17 P estradiol from their structure through the action of the esterase enzyme in the liver.

The biggest difference between these compounds is the half-life after administration. The duration of the half-life is greater in ascending order: E2, BE, VE and CE. The administration of a single injection of VE (5 mg) results in an increase in the plasma concentration of oestradiol for a period of five to seven days (BÓ et al., 1993), while a single injection of E2 (5 mg) results in an increase in the plasma concentration of oestradiol for only 42 hours. All the different types of oestradiol esters, including BE, VE and CE are capable of inducing the regression of antral follicles when administered in the presence of high concentrations of progesterone (BÓ et al., 1995).

2.5.3 Prostaglandin

Prostaglandins (PG), like leukotrienes and thromboxanes, are molecules derived from arachidonic and linoleic acids. The effects of the different prostaglandins (PGF_{2a}) on the reproduction of domestic animals are wide-ranging and can act on follicular development, ovulation, luteal regression, implantation and the maintenance of pregnancy, labour and puerperal physiology (WEEMS et al., 2005). PGF_{2a} and its synthetic analogues are used to synchronise the estrous cycle in domestic females due to their luteolytic action, which promotes vasoconstriction followed by an apoptotic cascade. PGF_{2a} and its analogues have therefore been the most widely used pharmacological agents in oestrus synchronisation programmes for bovine females (ODDE, 1990) and can be used alone or in combination with other hormones (THATCHER et al., 2002).

The success of the treatment depends on the presence of a CL, since the action of luteolin is to cause the morphological and functional regression of this structure (RATHBONE et al., 2001) and, consequently, a drop in endogenous progesterone concentrations. This is followed by an increase in gonadotrophin secretion and eventual ovulation. The drop in progesterone concentrations is rapid. Thus, fertility in these cases is equivalent to that of a spontaneous oestrus, since hormone concentrations (progesterone, oestrogen and LH) are basically the same as those found in untreated animals.

In females, with the lysis of the corpus luteum, oestrus appears at intervals of five or more days, which makes it impractical in IATF programmes (BÓ et al., 2002). This variation in the interval between the application of PGF_{2a} to oestrus and ovulation is due to the state of development of the follicles at the time of treatment (MARTINEZ et al., 2003). Thus, if the treatment is carried out when the dominant follicle is in the final phase of its growth, or at the beginning of its static phase, ovulation will occur within two to three days. On the other hand, if PGF_{2a} is applied when the dominant follicle is in the middle or end of its static phase, ovulation will occur five to seven days later, after the growth of the dominant follicle of the next follicular wave (KASTELIC and GINTHER, 1991). In this context, it should also be remembered that treatments carried out up to day 5 of the oestrus cycle (non-mature CL) do not effectively induce luteolysis (PARFET et al., 1989).

According to Wiltbank et al. (1975), there are some limitations to the use of prostaglandin. Firstly, the initial CL does not respond to treatment with the hormone, which can be solved by applying a second dose of PGF_{2a} with an interval that allows all females to present a responsive and functional CL. The recommended interval is 10 to 14 days. Secondly, PGF_{2a} does not induce oestrus in acyclic cows. Thirdly, females manifest oestrus at varying times shortly after treatment. This variability in the period of oestrus, as mentioned above, is due to differences between females in follicular growth, and not to differences in the period of luteal regression.

Theoretically, two applications of prostaglandin, at intervals of 11 to 14 days, induce oestrus in most cycling females, while females in oestrus or cycling irregularly do not respond to the treatment. In this sense, such programmes do not always provide a high degree of synchronisation or a high pregnancy rate (BARROS, 2000).

However, even after the application of 2 doses of PGF_{2a} , great variation has been observed in the detection of oestrus and ovulation in both *Bos taurus* and *Bos indicus*. This indicates that treatment with PGF_{2a} efficiently synchronises the moment of luteolysis and not the stage of development of the ovulatory follicle. Therefore, IATF protocols using prostaglandin alone have not shown good results. It is therefore necessary to use methods that control luteal and follicular development in order to synchronise follicle growth and ovulation.

2.5.4 Gonadotropin Releasing Hormone

Gonadotropin-releasing hormone (GnRH) is a decapeptide produced in the hypothalamus. This hypothalamic hormone is released in a pulsatile manner and, in the female, its frequency and amplitude vary during the reproductive stages in different species. LH synthesis and release are much more responsive to GnRH than FSH synthesis and release (VALLE et al., 1991; SANTOS, 2002).

The administration of GnRH raises the concentration of LH in the peripheral circulation over a period of 2 to 4 hours (TWAGIRAMUNGU et al., 1995). GnRH promotes ovulation or luteinisation of the dominant follicle if it is in its growth phase or at the beginning of its static phase (MARTINEZ et al., 2002), which results in the emergence of a new follicular wave.

Oestrus synchronisation protocols that use GnRH to initiate a new wave of follicle growth, or mainly to promote ovulation of a dominant follicle at the time of AI (or before), have been developed for beef and dairy cattle. In this sense, when administered at random stages of the oestrus cycle, GnRH can stimulate ovulation of the dominant follicle when it is larger than 9 mm, or atresia when it is smaller than 9 mm, and can induce the emergence of a new wave of follicular growth within 2 to 3 and/or 1 to 2 days in cows and heifers, respectively, after treatment (BRAGANÇA et al., 2007).

Alterations to the chemical structure of the natural GnRH molecule have led to the development of potent analogues (THATCHER et al., 2002). These include buserelin, gonadorelin and fertirelin acetate. Analogues stabilise the molecule against enzymatic attack, increase binding to plasma membranes and proteins, and increase the agonist's affinity for the GnRH receptor (THATCHER et al., 1993). Furthermore, they have a longer half-life in the circulation. These properties mean that the analogues can be used in lower doses than the natural form (D' OCCHIO et al., 1990).

In this sense, both buserelin acetate and gonadorelin diacetate are used to synchronise follicular waves and select dominant follicles at any time during the oestrus cycle and also to synchronise ovulation in IATF protocols (TWAGIRAMUNGU et al., 1995).

2.5.5 Equine Chorionic Gonadotropin

Equine chorionic gonadotrophin (eCG), also known as pregnant mare serum gonadotrophin (PMSG), is a glycoprotein produced by the endometrial calyces of mares between 40 and 120 days of pregnancy (GINTHER, 1979).

Compared to other gonadotrophic hormones, eCG is unique in that it has follicle stimulating and luteinising activity in the same molecule (PAPKOFF, 1974). Due to its dual action (as FSH and LH), eCG acts by directly stimulating follicular development and ovulation. The progesterone implant inhibits their release by the pituitary gland, reducing follicular development and ovulation until the desired time. When the implant is removed, the concentration of serum progesterone drops rapidly and the animal goes into oestrus. The administration of eCG in this case stimulates follicular development and enhances the synchronising action of progestogens. This is important given that the average diameter of postpartum follicles is smaller and they suffer atresia before reaching the ideal size to ovulate (MURPHY et al., 1990; YAVAS and WALTON, 2000).

When eCG is applied before progestogen withdrawal and in low doses, the dominant follicle becomes larger after progestogen treatment is suspended (LOGUÉRCIO, 2005). This increase in size probably leads to an improvement in pregnancy rates by stimulating greater development of the corpus luteum.

Based on these and other subsequent studies, and also on the properties of eCG, such as creating conditions for follicle growth and ovulation, it is clear that this substance is now being used in synchronisation and/or oestrus induction programmes in various species. Its use has proved rewarding in herds with a low cyclicity rate, such as in females with a postpartum period of less than 2 months and/or low body condition (BARUSELLI et al., 2004; DUFFY et al., 2004), as well as in pre-pubertal and pubertal heifers (BRANDÃO and SILVA FILHO, 2005).

The addition of eCG at the time of removal of the progesterone implant, using different progestogens, is an alternative for increasing pregnancy rates in IATF programmes with cows in anestrus or with low body condition (BÓ et al., 2003; BARUSELLI et al., 2004; BÓ et al., 2004).

3. FINAL CONSIDERATIONS

The estrous cycle of the female bovine is controlled by various intrinsic and extrinsic factors that directly affect the follicular dynamics of these animals and consequently reproduction and zootechnical indices. A better understanding of these factors is necessary in order to interfere in the management of these animals and thus obtain better reproductive rates and, consequently, more profitable cattle farming.

With the use of IATF, a significant improvement is expected in the pregnancy rates obtained from the correct use of hormones. This improvement reduces the calving interval between cows and increases the number of offspring per animal, as well as favouring general, health and nutritional management and promoting the genetic improvement of the herd, which is of fundamental importance for increasing productivity.

When choosing the IATF protocol to be used by the producer, the individual conditions of each herd must be analysed, as well as the cost/benefit ratio of its use.

4. REFERENCES

ALMERAYA, A. P. Reproductive Management in Cattle in Milk Production Systems. Faculty of Veterinary Medicine and Animal Science, National Autonomous University of Mexico, 2010.

ANUALPEC 2004. Brazilian Livestock Yearbook. FNP Consultoria & Agroinformativos. São Paulo: Topal & Comercial Biassi. Editora Gráfica, 2004. 376 p.

ARIAS, L. A. Q.; PABLO, C. D.; HERRADÓN, P. J. G.; MARTÍNEZ, A. I. P.; GONZÁLEZ, J. J. B. Ecografía y Reproducción en la Vaca, University of Santiago de Compostela, 2006.

Brazilian Artificial Insemination Association - ASBIA. Statistical report on semen production, imports and commercialisation, 2009. Available at . Accessed on 20 May 2016.

ASSIS, A. G.; STOCK, L.A.; CAMPOS, O.F.; GOMES, A.T.; ZOCCAL, R.; SILVA, M.R. Milk production systems in Brazil. Juiz de Fora: Embrapa Gado de Leite, 2005. 6p.

BANOS, G.; BROTHERSTONE, S.; COFFEY, M. P. Evaluation of body condition score measured throughout lactation as an indicator of fertility in dairy cows. Journal of Dairy Science. V. 87, p. 2669-2676, 2004.

BARBOSA, C.F.; JACOMINI J.O.; DINIZ, E.G. et al. Fixed-time artificial insemination and early pregnancy diagnosis in crossbred dairy cows. Revista Brasileira de Zootecnia, v.40, p. 79-84, 2011.

BARBOSA, C. F. [Fixed-time artificial insemination and pregnancy diagnosis in crossbred dairy cows]. 2009. 40 p. Dissertation (Master's) - Federal University of Uberlândia, Minas Gerais, 2009.

BARROS, C.M.; et al. Embryo transfer in *Bos indicus* cattle. Thereogenology. v. 56, p. 1483 - 1446, 2001.

BARROS, C.M.; MOREIRA, M.B.P.; FIGUEIREDO, R.A. et al. Synchronisation of ovulation in beef cows (*Bos indicus}* using GnRH, PGF2a and estradiol benzoate. Theriogenology, v.53, n.5, p.1121-1134, 2000.

BARUSELLI, P.S.; MADUREIRA, E.H. Symposium on pharmacological control of the estrous cycle in ruminants. São Paulo: Fundação da Faculdade de Medicina Veterinária e Zootecnia, USP, p. 332, 2000.

BARUSELLI, P. S.; SENEDA, M., Biotecnologia da Reprodução em Bovinos. 1. ed. São Paulo, v. 1, p. 246, 2004.

BARUSELLI, P. S.; MADUREIRA, E. H.; SÁ FILHO, M.F. et al. Effect of eCG treatment according to body condition score on conception rate of Nelore cows inseminated at fixed time. Acta Scientiae Veterinarie, v.32, p. 228, 2004.

BARUSELLI, P. S.; et al. Compendium of Animal Reproduction, Intervet, 399p. 2007.

BÓ, G.A.; ADAMS, G.P.; NASSER, L.F. et al. Effect of estradiol valerate on ovarian follicles, emergence of follicar waves and circulating gonadotropins in heifers. Theriogenology, v.40, p.225- 239, 1993.

BÓ, G.A.; ADAMS, G.P.; CACCIA, M. et al. Ovarian follicular wave emergence after treatment with progestagen and estradiol in cattle. Animal of Reproduction Science, v.39, p.193-204, 1995.

BÓ, G. A.; BROGLIATTI, G. M.; PIERSON, R. A. et al. Local versus systemic effect of exogenous estradiol-170 on ovarian follicular dynamics in heifers with progestogen implants. Animal Reproduction Science, v. 59, p. 141-157, 2000.

BÓ, G.A.; BARUSELLI, P.S.; MORENO, D. et al. The control of follicular wave development for self-appointed embryo transfer programmes in cattle. Theriogenology, v.57, p.53-72. 2002.

BÓ, G.A.; BARUSELLI, P.S.; MARTINEZ, M.F. Pattern and manipulation of follicular development in *Bos indicus*. Animal Reproduction Science, v.78, p.307-326, 2003.

BÓ, G.A.; CUTAIA, I.; BARUSELLI, P.S. Programas de inseminacion artificial y transferência de embriones a tiempofijo. In: INTERNATIONAL SYMPOSIUM ON APPLIED ANIMAL REPRODUCTION, 1st, 2004, São Paulo: FMZU - USP, p.56-80, 2004.

BRAGANÇA, J.F.M.; GONÇALVES, P.B.D.; BASTOS, G.M.; NEVES J.P.; OLIVEIRA J.F.C.; SIQUEIRA L.C.; BORGES L.F.K.; POMBO R.D. Synchronisation of oestrus and ovulation in heifers aged 12 to 14 months and artificially inseminated with oestrus observation and a pre-set schedule. Revista Brasileira de Reprodução Animal, v.28, n.2, p.73-77, 2004.

BRANDÃO, F.Z.; SILVA FILHO, J.M. Postpartum oestrus induction in primiparous Holstein-Zebu cows. Arquivo Brasileiro de Medicina Veterinária e Zootecnia, v.57, n.4, p.476-484, 2005.

BURKE, C. R.; MUSSARD, M. L.; GRUM, D. E. et al. Effects of maturity of the potential ovulatory follicle on induction of oestrus and ovulation in cattle with oestradiol benzoate. Animal Reproduction Science, v.66, p.161-174, 2001.

CASTILHO, C.; GAMBINI, A.L.C.; FERNANDES, P.; TRINCA, L.A.; TEIXEIRA, A.B.; BARROS, C.M. Synchronisation of ovulation in crossbred dairy heifers using gonadotrophin- releasing hormone agonist, prostaglandin F2a and human chorionic gonadotrophin or estradiol benzoate. Brazilian Journal of Medical and Biological Research, v. 33, p.91 - 101, 2000.

CHEBEL, R.C.; et al. Effect of fat sources differing in fatty acid profile on fertilisation rate and embryo quality in lactating dairy cows. Journal of Animal Science, v.82, p. 586, 2004.

CHRISTIAN. R.E; CASIDA.L.E. The effect of progesterone in altering the oestrual cycle of the cow. Journal of Animal Science, v.7, p.540, 1948.

CLARKE, J.J. GnRH secretion. In: International Congress On Animal Reproduction and Artificial Insemination, 5, 1988, Dublin. Proceedings...Dublin, p.1-9, 1988.

CUSTER E.E.; BEAL, W.E.; WILSON, S.J. et al. Effect of melengestrol acetate (MGA) or progesterone- releasing intravaginal device (PRID) on follicular development, concentrations of estradiol-17_ and progesterone, and LH release during an artificially lengthened bovine estrous cycle. Journal of Animal Science, v.72, p.1282-1289, 1994.

CUTAIA, L., TRIBULO, R., MORENO, D., BÓ, G.A. Pregnancy rates in lactating beef cows treated with progesterone releasing devices, estradiol and equine chorionic gonadotropin (eCG). Theriogenology, v. 59, p. 216, 2003.

DEMÉTRIO, D. G. B.; RODRIGUES, C. A.; SANTOS, R. M.; DEMÉTRIO, C. G. B.; CHIARI, J. R.; VASCONCELOS, J. L. M. Factors affecting conception rates following artificial insemination or embryo transfer in lactating Holstein cows. Journal of Dairy Science, v. 90, p. 5073 - 5082, 2007.

DUFFY, P.; CROWE, M.A.; AUSTIN, E.J. et al. The effect of eCG or estradiol at or after norgestomet removal on follicular dynamics, estrus and ovulation in early post-partum beef cows nursing calves. Theriogenology, v.61, p.725-734, 2004.

EMBRAPA GADO DE LEITE. Database. Available at: <http://www.cnpgl.embrapa.br/nova/informacoes/estatisticas/producao/tabela0240.php> Prepared by: R. ZOCCAL, 2006; accessed on 05 June 2012.

FERREIRA, A. M., Interaction between Nutrition and Reproduction: Reproductive Management of Females in the Tropics. Anais II Simpósio de Produção de Gado de Corte, p. 137-146, 2000.

FIKE, K.E.; DAY, M.L.; INSKEEP, E.K. et al. Estrus and luteal function in suckled beef cows that were anestrous when treated with an intravaginal device containing progesterone with or without a subsequent injection of estradiol benzoate. Journal of Animal Science, v.75, p.2009- 2015, 1997.

GIMENES, L. U; SÁ FILHO, M. F.; CARVALHO, N. A. T.; TORRES-JUNIOR, J. R. S.; SOUZA, A. H.; MADUREIRA, E. H.; TRINCA, L. A.; SARTORELLI, E. S.; BARROS, C. M.; CARVALHO, J. B. P.; MAPLETOFT, R. J.; BARUSELLI, P. S. Follicle deviation and ovulatory capacity in Bos indicus heifers. Theriogenology, v. 69, p. 852-858, 2008.

GINTHER, O. J.; BEG, M. A.; DONADEU, F. X.; BERGFELT, D. R. Mechanism of follicle deviation in monovular farm species. Animal Reproduction Science, v.78, p.239-257, 2003.

GINTHER, O.J. Influence of progesterone and number of corpora lutea on ovaries in sheep. American Journal of Veterinary Research, v.32, p.1987-1992, 1979.

GOTTSCHALL, C.S.; ALMEIDA, M.R.; TOLOTTI, F. et al. Evaluation of the reproductive performance of lactating beef cows submitted to IATF from the application of GnRH, oestrus manifestation, the reuse of... Acta ScientiaeVeterinariae. v.40, n.1, p. 1012. 2012.

GOUFERT, L.; et all. Fixed-time artificial insemination (FTAI) programmes. technical and economic aspects. EMBRAPA Cattle Reproduction Symposium, v. 1, p. 41-47, 2008.

GROHN, Y. T.; RAJALA - SCHULTZ, P. J. Epidemiology of reproductive performance in dairy cows. Animal Reproduction Science, v. 60 - 61, p. 6505 - 6514, 2000.

HAFEZ, E. S. E.; HAFEZ, B. Animal Reproduction. 7ª ed, Ed Manole LTDA, 530p, 2003.

HANSEN, P. J.; ARECHIGA, C. F. Strategies for managing reproduction in heat-stressed dairy cows. Journal of Animal Science, v. 77, suppl. 2, p. 36-50, 2000.

BRAZILIAN INSTITUTE OF GEOGRAPHY AND STATISTICS. Aggregated data bank. Available at : <http://www.ibge.gov.br/estadosat/temas.php?sigla=es&tema=pecuaria2011>. Accessed on: 04 May 2013.

KASTELIC, J.P.; GINTHER, O.J. Factors affecting the origin of the ovulatory follicle in heifers with induced luteolysis. Animal of Reproduction Science, v.26, n.1-2, p.13-24, 1991.

KESNER, J.S.; PADMANABHAN, V.; CONVEY, E.M. Estradiol induces and progesterone inhibits the preovulatory surges of luteinising hormone and folliclestimulating hormone in heifers. Biology of Reproduction, v.26, p.571-578, 1982.

KINDER J.E. Frequency of luteinising hormone pulses and circulating 170-oestradiol concentration in cows is related to concentration of progesterone comes from Esther in endogenous or exogenous source. Animal of Reproduction Science, v.37, p.257-265, 1996.

LARSON, L.L.; BALL, P.J.H. Regulation of estrus cycle in dairy cattle: a review. Theriogenology, v.38, p.255-267, 1992.

LOGUÉRCIO, R.S. Regulation of steroid receptors and follicular dynamics in a postpartum hormone induction system in beef cows. 80f. Thesis (Doctorate in Veterinary Medicine), Postgraduate Course in Veterinary Medicine, Federal University of Santa Maria, Santa Maria, 2005.

LOPEZ-GATIUS, F.; SANTOLARIA, P.; MARTINO, A. et al. The effects of GnRH treatment at the time of AI and 12 days later on reproductive performance of high producing dairy cows during the warm season in northeastern Spain. Theriogenology, v. 65, p. 820-830, 2006.

MACIEL, A. B. DE B. A proposal for assessing body condition in Holstein and Nelore cows. 2006. 103 p. Dissertation (Master's in Zootechnics) - Faculty of Veterinary Medicine and Zootechnics, Universidade Estadual Paulista, Botucatu, SP.

MADUREIRA, E.H.; BARUSELLI, P.S.; MARQUES, M.O. Pharmacological Control of the Estrus Cycle in Ruminants. 1.ed. São Paulo: Fundação da Faculdade de Medicina Veterinária e Zootecnia / USP, v.1, p.89-98, 2009.

MARTINEZ, M.F.; KASTELIC, J.P.; ADAMS, G.P. et al. The use of progestins in regimens for fixed-time artificial insemination if beef cattle. Theriogenology, v.57, p.1049-1059, 2002.

MARTINEZ, M.F.; KASTELIC, J.P.; COLAZO, M.G. Effects of estradiol on gonadotrophin release, estrus and ovulation in CIDR-treated beef cattle. Domes anim. Endocrinologist, v.33. p.77 - 90, 2003.

MENEGHETTI, M.; SÁ FILHO, O.G.; PERES, R.F.G. et al. Fixed-time artificial insemination with estradiol and progesterone for *Bos indicus* cows I: Basis for development of protocols. Theriogenology, v.72, p.179-189, 2009.

MENEGHETTI, M.; VASCONCELOS, J. L. M. Calving month, body condition and response to fixed-time artificial insemination protocol in primiparous beef cows. Arquivo Brasileiro de Medicina Veterinária e Zootecnia, Belo Horizonte, v. 60, n. 4, p. 786-793, 2008.

MIHM, M.; AUSTIN, E.J. Effect of duration of dominance of the ovulatory follicle on onset of estrus and fertility in heifers. Journal of Animal Science, v.77, p.2219-2226. 2002.

MONTEZUMA JR, P. A. [Postpartum reproductive performance of mixed-breed dairy cows (3/8 Holandês X 5/8 Gir) submitted to a hormonal treatment based on GnRH and prostaglandin F2a]. 2001. 70 p. Dissertation (Master's Degree) - Federal University of Ceará, Fortaleza, 2001.

MONTIEL, F.; AHUJA, C. Body condition and suckling as factors influencing the duration of postpartum anestrus in cattle: a review. Animal Reproduction Science, v. 85, p. 1-26, 2005.

MORAES, J.C.F.; SOUZA, C.J.H.; GONCALVES, P.B.D. et al. Control of oestrus and ovulation in cattle and sheep. In: GONCALVES, P.B.D; FIGUEIREDO, J.R; FREITAS, V.J. Biotécnicas Aplicadas à Reprodução Animal. São Paulo: Livraria Varela, Chap.2, p.25-55, 2001.

MURPHY, M.G.; BOLAND, M.P.; ROCHE, J.F. Pattern of follicular growth and resumption of ovarian activity in post-partum beef suckler cows. Journal of Reproduction and Fertility, v.90, n.2, p.523-533.1990.

NEVES, J.P.; MIRANDA, K.L.; TORTORELLA, R.D. Scientific progress in reproduction in the first decade of the 21st century. Revista Brasileira de Zootecnia, v. 39, p. 414-421, 2010.

ODDE, K.G. A review of synchronisation of estrus in postpartum cattle. Journal of Animal Science, v.68, n.3, p.817-830, 1990.

PAPKOFF, H. Chemical and properties of the subunits of pregnant mare serum gonadotropin. Biochemical and Biophysical Research Communications, v.58, n.2, p.397-404, 1974.

PARFET, J.R. Secretory patterns of LH and FSH and follicular growth following administration of PGF2a during the early luteal phase in cattle. Theriogenology, v.31, n.3, p.513-524, 1989.

RATHBONE, M.J.; KINDER, J.E.; FIKE, K. et al. Recent advances in bovine reproductive endocrinology and physiology and their impact on drug delivery system design for the control of the estrous cycle in cattle. Advance Drug Delivery Reviews, v.50, n.3, p.277-320, 2001.

REVAH, I.; BUTLER, W.R. Prolonged dominance of follicles and reduced viability of bovine oocytes. Journal of Reproduction and Fertility, v.106, n.1, p.39-47, 1996.

SÁ FILHO, O. G.; DIAS, C. C.; VASCONCELOS, J. L. M. Effect of progesterone or 17p - estradiol on luteal lifespan in anoestrous Nelore cows. Journal Animal Science, v. 84, suppl. 1, p. 207 (Abstract), 2006.

SANTOS, M.D.; VASCONCELOS, J.L.M.; PEREZ, G.C. et al. Oestrus percentage and pregnancy rate of Nelore cows synchronised with CIDR-B. Revista Brasileira de Reprodução Animal, v.25, n.3, p.308- 310, 2002.

SARTORI, R., FRICKE, P. M., FERREIRA, J. C. et al. Follicular deviation and acquisition of ovulatory capacity in bovine follicles. Biology Reproduction, v.65, p.1403-1409, 2001.

SARTORI, R. Reproductive management of the dairy female. Revista Brasileira de Reprodução Animal, Belo Horizonte, v. 31, n. 2, p. 153 - 159, 2007.

SENGER, P. L. Pathways to Pregnancy and Parturition, 2ª ed, Ed Current Conceptions, Washington, 2003.

SEVERO, N. C. Impact of artificial insemination on the cattle industry in Brazil and worldwide. Revista Veterinária e Zootecnia em Minas, 2009.

SHELDON, I. M.; NOAKES, D. E.; DOBSON, H. The influence of ovarian activity and uterine involution determined by ultrasonography on subsequent reproductive performance of dairy cows. Theriogenology, v. 54, p. 409-419, 2000.

SIQUEIRA, L.C.; OLIVEIRA, J.F.C.; LOGUÉRCIO, R.S. et al. Two-day or fixed-time artificial insemination systems for lactating cows. Ciência Rural, v.38, n.2, p.411- 415. 2008.

SOUZA, A.H.; SILVA, E.P.B.; CUNHA, A.P. et al. Ultrasonographic evaluation of endometrial thickness near timed AI as a predictor of fertility in high-producing dairy cows. Theriogenology, v.75, p.722-33, 2011.

STUMPF, T.T.; DAY, M.L.; WOLFE, M.W. et al. Effect of estradiol on luteinizing hormone secretion during the follicular phase of the bovine estrous cycle. Biology of Reproduction, v.41, p.91-99, 1989.

THATCHER, W.W.; DROST, M.; SAVIO, J.D. et al. New clinical uses of GnRH and its analogues in cattle. Animal of Reproduction Science, v.33, p.27-49, 1993.

THATCHER, W.W.; MOREIRA, F.; PANCARCIA, S.M. et al. Strategies to optimise reproductive efficiency by regulation of ovarian function. Domestic Animal Endocrinology, v.23, p.243-254, 2002.

THATCHER, W.W.; MOREIRA F.; SANTOS J.E.P.; MATTOS R.C.; LOPES F.L.; PANCARCI S.M.; RISCO C.A. Effects of hormonal treatments on reproductive performance and embryo production. Theriogenology, v.25, p. 75 - 89, 2001.

TWAGIRAMUNGU, H.; GUILBAULT, L.A.; DUFOUR, J.J. Synchronisation of ovarian follicular waves with a gonadotropin-releasing hormone agonist to increase the precision of estrus in cattle: a review. Journal of Animal Science, v.73, p.3141-3151, 1995.

VALLE, E.R.; ENCARNAÇÃO, R.O.; PADOVANI, C.R. Estrous behaviour and the estrus-to-ovulation interval in Nelore cattle *(Bos indicus)* with natural estrus or estrus induced with prostaglandin F2alpha or norgestomet and estradiol valerate. Theriogenology, v.49, p.667-681, 1991.

VOGG, G.; SOUZA, C.J.H.; JAUME, C.M.; MORAES J.C.F. Usefulness of oestradiol benzoate after progestogen supplementation in oestrus synchronisation of beef heifers. Acta Scientiae Veterinariae, v.32, p. 41 - 46, 2004.

WEEMS, C.W.; WEEMS, Y.S.; RANDEL, R.D. Prostaglandins and reproduction in females farm animals. The Veterinary Journal, v.171, p.206-228, 2005.

WILTBANK, M. C.; GÜMEN, A.; SARTORI, R. Physiological classification of anovulatory conditions in cattle. Theriogenology, v. 57, p. 21 - 52, 2002.

WILTIBANK, M.C.; LOPEZ, H.; SARTORI, R. et al. Changes in reproductive physiology of lactating dairy cows due to elevated steroid metabolism. Theriogenology, v. 65, p, 17-29, 2006.

WILTBANK, M.C. How information on hormonal regulation of the ovary has improved understanding of timed breeding programmes. Proceedings Annual Meeting Society For Theriogenology, p.83-97, 1975.

WOAD, D.G.; ARMSTRONG, D.G. Corpus luteum (CL) function: local control mechanisms. Domestic Animal Endocrinology, v.5339, p.1-9, 2002.

YAVAS, Y; WALTON, J.S. Induction of ovulation in postpartum suckled beef cows: a review. Theriogenology, v.54, p.1-23, 2000.

ZANCHET, E. Effect of two prostaglandin F2a injections after calving on reproductive performance of dairy cows and reproductive efficiency between Holstein and Jersey breeds. A Hora Veterinária, n. 143, p. 13-17, 2005.

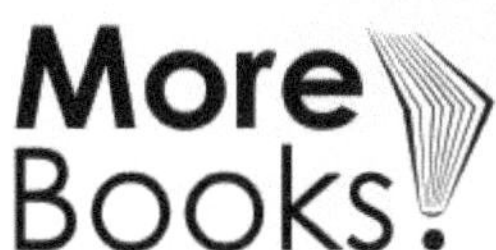

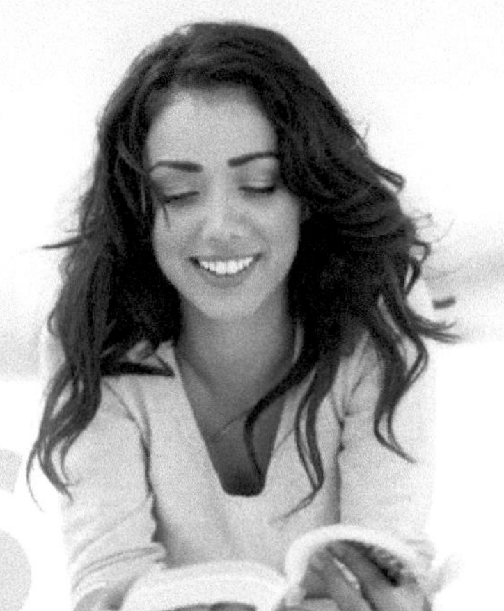

yes I want morebooks!

Buy your books fast and straightforward online - at one of world's fastest growing online book stores! Environmentally sound due to Print-on-Demand technologies.

Buy your books online at
www.morebooks.shop

Kaufen Sie Ihre Bücher schnell und unkompliziert online – auf einer der am schnellsten wachsenden Buchhandelsplattformen weltweit! Dank Print-On-Demand umwelt- und ressourcenschonend produziert.

Bücher schneller online kaufen
www.morebooks.shop

info@omniscriptum.com
www.omniscriptum.com

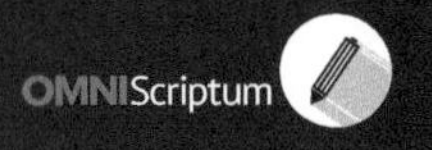

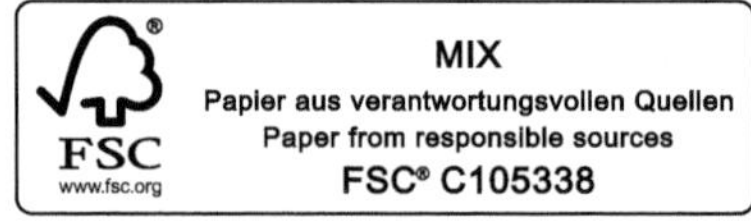

Printed by Books on Demand GmbH, Norderstedt / Germany